SUGAR DETOX

A Nutritionist's Guide to Crush Carb Cravings, Lose Weight & Reduce Inflammation - Simple Tips & Recipes to Take Back Your Health

SIMON KELLER

© **Copyright 2018 – (Simon Keller) All rights reserved.**

The contents of this book may not be reproduced, duplicated or transmitted without direct written permission from the author. Under no circumstances will any legal responsibility or blame be held against the publisher for any reparation, damages, or monetary loss due to the information herein, either directly or indirectly.

Legal Notice:

This book is copyright protected. This is only for personal use. You cannot amend, distribute, sell, use, quote or paraphrase any part or the content within this book without the consent of the author.

Disclaimer Notice:

Please note the information contained within this document is for educational and entertainment purposes only. Every attempt has been made to provide accurate, up to date and reliable complete information. No warranties of any kind are expressed or implied. Readers acknowledge that the author is not engaging in the rendering of legal, financial, medical or professional advice. The content of this book has been derived from various sources. Please consult a licensed professional before attempting any techniques outlined in this book.

By reading this document, the reader agrees that under no circumstances are is the author responsible for any losses, direct or indirect, which are incurred as a result of the use of information contained within this document, including, but not limited to, —errors, omissions, or inaccuracies.

TABLE OF CONTENTS

Part 1: A Scientific & Historical Overview of Sugar....7

Chapter 1: The History of Sugar - How it Became so Prevalent in Society...9

Chapter 2: The Science of Sugar - A Necessary Evil........21

Chapter 3: Health Consequences of Consuming Too Much of the Sweet Stuff 35

Chapter 4: Humanities Drug of Choice - Are You Addicted? 45

Part 2: Practical Ways to Eliminate Added Sugar From Your Diet (and replace with healthier alternatives) 49

Chapter 5: Getting Off the Sugar Rush Roller Coaster! ..51

Chapter 6: Zero Sugar Recipes and Alternative Meal Plans...55

Chapter 7: Drinks & Beverages - The Easiest Way to Reduce Your Sugar Intake...................................63

Chapter 8: Mindsets & Habits - Overcoming Roadblocks to Sugar Free Success 69

Summary...77

Conclusion 81

INTRODUCTION

"Sugar is the sociopath of foods. It acts sweet…
but its really poison"

(Karen Salmansohn)

It's important to note that sugar is essential for our bodies. It's the substance which fuels all of our biological systems (brain, muscles, organs) in the form of glucose. Its the natural sugars found in fruits and starchy vegetables which most readily provide these energy substrates. Broken down from the carbohydrates in these whole foods, sugar is what drives us forward and keeps us operating optimally.

So why do so many people suffer the ill consequences of consuming sugar and benefit so greatly when detoxing from it? The answer is simple. It's the type and amount of sugar we consume in today's society which is the problem. More accurately, it's refined and processed sugar which is the problem. It's the "added sugar" which is the enemy here.

Combined with chemically laden processed foods and high saturated fat intake. High added sugar consumption is one of, if not the greatest driver of the ever increasing health issues we face today. Obesity and diabetes levels are at record highs across the world, and alarmingly this is no longer a problem confined to the West. Developing nations are quickly adopting a more "Standard American" diet and sadly the ailments and illnesses such eating habits provide.

You may have heard that everything in moderation is OK, and I agree with this to some degree. However most peoples idea of moderation is way off the mark. They believe that by eating the right things 50% of the time (every other meal) is sufficient to stay in good health. It is not. The data is pretty clear on this. The body has not nearly enough time to heal itself, reduce the inflammation and remove the toxins from such a high frequency of damaging food sources.

Others choose to moderate things with perhaps one "cheat day" a week in and 80-20 type fashion. Or better yet 90-10, where you are treating yourself to just one "cheat meal" a week, or 10% "bad" food sources to keep yourself sane. This can work well with fatty foods such as burgers and fries for instance. However, sugary foods are somewhat different due to the addictive nature of them. If you allow yourself to let just a little refined sweetness into your day, it can be a slippery slope. The next thing you know you are chomping down doughnuts and candy bars everyday! I know this one all too well…

From my experience going cold turkey on sugar (at least to begin with) is the best way to go, hence why I'm writing this book. You will find that it takes only 3-4 days for your taste buds and digestive system to get over the elimination of these foods. After this point, you will no longer crave them.

You will even find that your palate starts to become much more sensitive to these natural sources of sugar, fresh fruit, berry's, dates etc. They will become extremely sweet to the taste. The old adage that healthy food tastes bland and boring goes out of the window at this point. These foods actually begin to taste too sweet for some people!

Not only that, it becomes extremely easy to detect refined & added sugar in foods as well as artificial sweeteners. These "junk foods" will simply not taste like food anymore, just a sickly sweetened and salty mess. Even the more "natural" added sugars such as honey, maple syrup and brown sugar will taste like overkill for you.

There are so many benefits which come from cutting out this sweet little devil in your diet. Your health and well-being will improve immeasurably if you can successfully kick this habit. It's certainly not easy, but there honestly isn't a wiser investment you can make for your future than performing a continuing sugar detox. My aim for this book is to walk you through the steps on exactly how to do it!

SIMON KELLER

My Credentials

Before we get into the nitty-gritty of sugar detoxing, it's probably a good idea for me to explain exactly who I am, and why you should even bother listening to me in the first place. Yes I have the undergraduate in anatomy and physiology, and the master's degree in nutrition from Birmingham University in the UK.

However my main focus over the past 10 years has been on the practical implications of human performance. I now focus much more on the results of these principles in the real world, compared to my previous life of studying endless research papers on the academic side of the subject.

This includes everything from human movement to dietary considerations. What set of variables is most optimal for both myself, and the clients I now coach and mentor within my specialized training and wellness complex here in London.

Not everyone is the same, however there is a surprising amount of overlap when it comes to human physiology. With a few minor age, gender and genetic variations aside, we are all working with pretty much the same metabolic machinery. You just need to know how to get the most from it.

So why am I such an expert on sugar detoxing? As I mentioned, I studied a wide range of topics within the field of cardiovascular/respiratory physiology and nutrition whilst at university. This formed my base understanding of these subjects and how they fit together within a biological sense.

However I have since put these academic theories and principles to the test in the real world. To really see what works and what doesn't with regards to completing the health and fitness puzzle. One of the biggest discoveries I've come to realize is our miss use of our essential fuel source, sugar.

I have undertook a journey of personal development and experimentation when it comes to human performance on myself first and foremost. I like to consider myself somewhat of a guinea pig when it comes to the physiological principles I test. I can then advise my clients on the best course of action for them. How we use the sweet stuff has been central to this research over the past 3 years.

The result of all this study has lead to me getting paid large sums to educate and train business professionals, athletes etc. However I still only have time to focus on a handful of clients at any one time. This is why I have switched to writing and publishing more work on these subjects, in order to educate as many people as I can, at a fraction of the cost of my one-on-one coaching.

Everything from devising peoples workout routines to managing their eating plans. From providing motivational and psychological guidance to lifestyle tips. I like to provide everything as a holistic approach to human performance. Because lets face it, we don't live out our lives in nice compartmentalized boxes. Everything blends into one, you have to up your efforts across the board to reap the full benefits of a healthy body and mind.

What I have come to find is that radically changing our use of the most addictive dietary substance (refined sugar) plays a major role in fixing many of the human aliments we face today. Health, mood regulation, improved sleep… the list goes on.

The following chapters will teach you everything you need to know about performing a successful sugar detox. The theories behind the science, and how you can best implement them practically into your own life, to garner the amazing results that reducing or eradicating this substance from your diet can bring. This is one adjustment you can make which will have a big difference in your life. So get ready to give this a try, I promise you it will be worth it.

PART 1: A SCIENTIFIC & HISTORICAL OVERVIEW OF SUGAR

CHAPTER 1: THE HISTORY OF SUGAR - HOW IT BECAME SO PREVALENT IN SOCIETY

Sugar use has been a staple part of the human experience for such a long time now that we almost take it for granted. No modern home is void of at least of few bags in the kitchen cupboards at any one time. After all, how do you sweeten your dishes without it right? How would your coffee taste without a spoonful or two? How would you bake cakes and pastries without the white stuff?

As you load some sugar packs into your grocery cart each week, have you ever wondered about its origins? Who discovered sugar and when did mankind start using it to sweeten their food in such a widespread manner? Was sugar always such an essential additive as it is today?

In order to know this we need to understand the history of sugar. To investigate its background and the roles sugar has played in the lives of our ancestors. Only then will it be possible to realize the full extent of its impact on society. Both the positive and negative effects it has brought to our lives today.

Sweet Beginnings – Sugar's First Discovery

The discovery of sugar in its raw form I.e. via extraction from the sugarcane plant, was made by the Polynesians who lived in Papua New Guinea around 8,000 BC. Researchers widely believed that sugarcane domestication and cultivation occurred alongside other important crops such as the banana and taro during this time.

Sugar was not initially part of our ancestors' diet. Early man mostly consumed plant crops and animal meat they'd hunted and gathered from the lands in which they roamed. Some evidence points to these early humans using honey to sweeten their food, however not sugarcane extracts just yet.

It was very likely that they used sugarcane extracts to help fatten the pigs and other animals they were raising. But the discovery of sugar's sweet taste was probably made by accident, when humans also began to chew on sugarcane stalks when their own food supplies ran low.

From the Polynesians to the Indians

Sugarcane crops were carried by Polynesian seafarers across the Pacific and Indian oceans, helping spread sugarcane cultivation to places in Southeast Asia, China, and finally to India. The climatic conditions of India made it possible for the local populations to continue cultivating sugarcane plants on a large-scale basis. It was in India where the first organized mass sugar production started.

Initially, the Indians had to chew on the plant stalks first and foremost, in order to extract the sweet juice from cane sugar. However in 350AD, they developed a more efficient extraction process, wherein the crystallized white powder was extracted from the sugarcane plants. This marked the beginning of the introduction of sugar as a new "sweet spice" exclusively made by the Indians.

The creation of the first refined sugar source provided the locals the opportunity to gain extensive profits from its trade with neighbouring countries. Hence, Indians traded their refined cane sugar extensively with China, Persia, and other Middle Eastern countries. These trading activities helped spread the knowledge and use of this so-called "honey powder", as demands for cane sugar rose across the Middle Eastern area. Cane sugar, therefore, became a highly-valued commodity during this period.

The Medieval Islamic and Egyptian World

The Arab Agricultural Revolution (8th to 13th centuries) saw the improvement of sugar production greatly. Islamic scientists devised new presses which enabled them to extract more juices from the sugarcane plants compared with previous methods. This translated into larger amounts of sugar production and more importantly, even greater profits at the time.

During this period, the Arab nations began incorporating this sweet condiment into their cuisine. People from other lands were amazed by these edible sweet products from the Middle Easterners, driving their curiosity about sugar. Meanwhile, those in ancient Fatimid Egypt began trading sugar to Europeans in 1100 AD. As the demand for this new sweet commodity rose, these early Egyptians began to create water-mills to grind the sugar granules from its liquid form.

However, the incessant growth of this sweet substance sweeping the world wasn't without its set-backs. A decline in sugar sales occurred during the reign of the Mamluk government around 1300 AD. Sugar became much more expensive due to the Mamluk's improper means of successfully regulating the trading systems during this time. Hence, the Europeans who had been consistently purchasing sugar from Egyptians previously, were now forced to try growing sugar cane for themselves.

Sugar in Europe during the Middle Ages

Sugar cultivation and production didn't reach the Mediterranean region in earnest until the 13th century. The Crusaders returning home from their travels played a major role in ensuring that sugar was now commonplace in their European homelands. They often talked about this new "sweet spice", thus, elevating the status of sugar to a luxurious, rare, and expensive commodity item to trade.

As mentioned previously, Europeans began growing sugarcane plants partly as they grew tired of the exorbitant prices of Egyptian sugar under the Mamluk government. They found it difficult to grow the plant in Northern Europe. Hence, the cities of Sicily and Cyprus were used to cultivate the sugarcane plants primarily. Sugarcane was also grown in the Canary Islands and in the southern most regions of Spain.

Sugar and the Slave Trade

As the Europeans continued to develop sugar in the 14th and 15th centuries, the need for an ever larger workforce on the sugarcane farms and mills increased alongside this. Sugar production required intensive labor, so the Europeans began to consider the use of the slave trade to meet the requirements of this work. Hence, the increasing demand for sugar production helped pave the way for slavery in Europe.

This new workforce who labored the sugarcane farms and mills at the time, came primarily from areas around West Africa and the Black Sea. A wave of transatlantic migration flourished during this period as a result, with more than 13 million people being shipped to Europe and the Americas for this forced labor.

Vested European Interests in Sugar Production and Trade

Governments across the world saw the monetary potential which sugar production provided, and thus began to impose heavy taxes on cane sugar products. This is why sugar remained a luxury item, which the average citizen could still not afford during the 1700's to 1800's.

Worldwide interest in sugar never halted though as the 19th century set in. Many European countries still had vested interests in sugar production, as the demand was still high and the profits still lucrative. Britain blocked the continuing cane sugar trade to Europe at the onset of the Napoleonic wars. Continental Europe was then forced to find other sources of sugar to keep up with their demands.

The Entrance of Sugar Beets

In an effort to find ever cheaper alternatives to cane sugar, the king of Prussia (A German Empire at the time) offered support and finances to gain greater knowledge on sugar extraction. Answering this call, a German chemist named Andreas Sigismund Marggraf discovered another source of sugar in 1747 – which was the beet plant.

Marggraf and his students discovered that beetroots also contained sugar identical to that obtained from sugar cane plants. Due to this finding, efforts were made to develop sugar from beetroots across the land of Silesia (modern-day Poland). Factories were opened in Silesia, and the Silesian white sugar beet was soon introduced to North America and Chile in the mid-1800's. Beet sugar then became the main sugar source of the European continent during this time.

The Mechanization of Sugar Production

The 18th century saw the need for a reduction in manual labor, as the mechanization of sugar was slowly starting to take hold. The invention of the steam engine was a critical introduction to the sugar mills and a significant upgrade when it came to pulverizing the sugar cane plants. This breakthrough increased sugar production immensely, as the machines could essentially work 24 hours daily with just a little human supervision.

Other notable mechanization processes became prevalent during this time also, which included:

- The use of closed kettles in order to boil sugar yields for even more sugar granules. This was discovered by an English chemist named Edward Charles Howard in 1813.

- Evaporators were created by an American engineer, Norbert Rillieux, in 1820. This further improved the refining process.

- Utilizing a mechanical centrifuge to separate sugar from molasses was pioneered by David Weston, an American, in Hawaii not long after this.

Each of these advancements reduced the need for human labor in the sugar production and refinement process. This in turn aided the dissolution of slavery in the sugar cane plantations and simultaneously accelerated the production of sugar worldwide.

Affordable Sugar in Modern Times

As a result of these advancements in sugar technology, higher prices slowly declined as consumption continuously rose, whilst the mechanization of sugar production continuously improved. In fact the British Prime Minister at the time, William Ewart Gladstone, choose to abolish sugar tariffs altogether in 1874. This extensively brought down sugar prices within reach of the average British citizen.

Sugar became more affordable as mechanized production flourished all the more during the 1900's. The masses were finally able to get a taste of these sweet granules that were once confined to the higher classes who could afford it within continental Europe.

Competitors of Sugar in Today's World

Nowadays, both cane and beet sugar have met their competitors I.e. high-fructose corn syrups and artificial sweeteners. High fructose corn syrup was discovered by Earl P. Kooi and Richard O. Marshall in 1957; however, the product wasn't fully perfected until the 1970's.

This syrup was extracted from corn in an attempt to turn corn's glucose content into a sweeter fructose. Popularity of high-fructose corn syrup rose in the United States during the late 1970s as a result of an abundant supply of local corn and the skyrocketing prices of table sugar due to import taxes.

Artificial sweeteners also became popular alternatives to cane and beet sugar. The earliest known artificial sweetener was saccharin, discovered in 1878 by laboratory assistant Constantin Fahlberg. Other artificial sweeteners we see today include:

- Stevia
- Aspartame
- Sucralose
- Cyclamate, and
- Curculin

These artificial sweeteners became very popular as they are far cheaper to produce and synthesize compared with cane sugar. They also do not contain any calories, which is beneficial for those who are attempting to lose weight (even sugar detox). They cause less dental issues and are claimed to be generally better for diabetic patients. However they do not come without their own drawbacks and side effects which we will explore later on.

Where We Currently Stand on the White Stuff

Sugar has been used for just about every purpose over the centuries including medicinal purposes to alleviate human gastrointestinal problems and stomach illnesses alike. It has also been viewed as a valuable spice, preservative, and food sweetener. Eventually, sugar became a luxury item that only the wealthiest of the European gentry were able to consume.

Sugar's history has affected the world's development in such drastic ways. From the discovery and development of sugar in ancient times, all the way up to the present day. Everything from, human slavery, colonialism, exclusivity to the higher classes, vested monetary interests and political influences who dictated changes in sugar prices.

Today, the rise of high-fructose corn syrup and artificial sweeteners has not outshone the sugar demands and consumption's of modern civilization. Statistics even suggest that the world has consumed approximately 172 million metric tons of sugar during 2016 to 2017 alone.

Sugar is now a commodity, not a luxury. Almost every kitchen in the world keeps some form of table, cane, or beet sugar in their cupboards. Sugar approximately accounts for 20% of our modern day dietary calories. It's present in almost every food and drink you can think of, even in those which are not generally sweet. Although it does provide us an energy substrate, sugar itself isn't a nutritious substance, yet the world craves it. The advertisement industry certainly has played their part in this development too.

Foods with high added sugar content are constantly pushed onto us. They are advertised to the masses in an attempt to keep sugar demands high. Fast foods, chips, candies, cakes, pastries, artificial juices, and carbonated soft drinks all use lots of sugar in their production. These food products are extensively advertised and designed to keep us coming back for more.

This is all done in the face of the known health hazards of consuming too much sugar too. Governments continue to impose discreet worldwide taxes on the sweet stuff, all whilst populations suffer and environmental sacrifices which are required to cultivate sugar plants instead of more nutritious and sustainable food sources.

Sugar remains the dominating commodity in our life today, if we know it or not. This simple and sweet substance has indeed changed our world drastically over the centuries, and it's now time for this dependence to stop.

CHAPTER 2: THE SCIENCE OF SUGAR - A NECESSARY EVIL

Have you ever wondered what sugar is actually comprised of? Have you ever taken the time to stop and think about what's truly inside those sweet, small, white granules you use in your food every day? Most people would be surprised to know that sugar isn't made up of just one component, but many.

"Sugar" has a vast classification, and it's not simply limited to the table sugar we're all so familiar with. There are many types and they each affect our bodies in significantly different ways. It's time for a little science here. Let us explore the different types of sugar and how they work inside our bodies. The benefits this energy substrate brings, as well as the downsides excess amounts has on our health and well-being.

Defining Sugar Scientifically

We all know sugar's loose definition – those sweet-tasting white granules used to improve the flavor of many kinds of food. But scientifically, sugar isn't confined to that white stuff we often associate it with.

Sugar is essentially a type of carbohydrate, a macronutrient required by the body to sustain life. Sugar is a liquid-soluble organic compound which is derived from different food sources. One molecule of sugar contains varying amounts of carbon, hydrogen, and oxygen atoms.

Since sugar is a carbohydrate by nature, it gives off energy to the body when digested. However each form isn't created equal. Different types of sugar provide varying levels of energy to the body.

The Different Types of Sugar

Sugars can be classified into three main category types: monosaccharides, disaccharides, and polysaccharides.

1. Monosaccharides

Monosaccharides are the simplest forms of sugars which exist. They cannot be hydrolyzed or broken down into smaller molecules from their current form. This sugar type is also the basic form of carbohydrates. Monosaccharides often present themselves physically as colorless water-soluble crystals. Most of these compounds have a sweet taste.

Monosaccharides can be further divided into three different types:

A. Galactose – This is a simple sugar which differs slightly from glucose in its molecular structure. It is less sweet than fructose and glucose. Its physical form is an odor-free white crystalline powder.

It is synthesized by the body and is broken down into glucose during digestion. When combined with glucose, galactose forms another sugar type called lactose.

Galactose is present in milk, yogurt, cheese, and other dairy products.

B. Fructose – This simple sugar is widely known as the "fruit sugar" due to it's abundance within fruits and juices. It is commercially available in powder and syrup forms also.

This sugar is not an essential nutrient; you don't have to get your daily fix of fructose in order to stay healthy. But fructose still functions in the body to increase the absorption of potassium, sodium, and water.

Common fruit sources include mangoes, apples, watermelon, grapes, bananas, and dates. Fructose is also present in honey, high-fructose corn syrup, agave syrup, and carbonated soft drinks. More on this later.

C. Glucose – This is a simple sugar produced after the breakdown and digestion of carbohydrates in our bodies. Glucose carries the energy taken from digested food and distributes it to the various working cells of the body via the bloodstream.

Glucose is the only type of sugar which the brain can use to fuel cognition. Approximately 100-130 grams of glucose is required for the brain to function optimally on a daily basis. Glucose is also administered to patients with low blood sugar levels.

Dietary sources of natural glucose include fresh and dried fruits, honey, nuts, legumes, seeds, vegetables, and cereals. Glucose may also be added to foods artificially. Processed foods and fruit juices may carry artificial glucose, especially when the labels carry the name "dextrose".

2. Disaccharides

Disaccharides are simple sugars composed of a combination of two monosaccharides. They can still be broken down into smaller sugars. Like monosaccharides, disaccharides are also a form of simple carbohydrates.

Disaccharides are further classified into these three major types:

A. Sucrose – This is a disaccharide composed of fructose and glucose. Sucrose is more popularly known as table sugar, both the refined white sugar and the raw brown version.

Sucrose exists physically as the sugar we all know – white crystalline granules with a pleasantly sweet taste. Sucrose may also be found in syrup form. It can be a source of energy, but is not absolutely necessary that you consume it to stay energized and healthy.

This sugar type can be used to treat children with low blood sugar levels. Some also use it as an effective pain intervention for babies undergoing painful procedures.

Foods rich in natural sucrose include table sugar, beet sugar, date palm, and sorghum. Sucrose can also be found in commercially prepared food products such as syrup sweeteners, jams, sweet beverages, chewing gums, and candies.

B. Lactose – This disaccharide is a product of the combination of glucose and galactose. Lactose is widely known as milk sugar.

Lactose is broken down by the body through an enzyme called lactase. This enzyme is found in the small intestine. But some people have a lactase deficiency, making them unable to digest lactose properly.

Others may have adequate amounts of lactase, but their gastric tract becomes irritated once lactose is ingested and digestion begins. These people are said to be lactose-intolerant, which is much more prevalent than even most people would think.

Abundant food sources which contain lactose include milk, infant formula, ice cream, yogurt, and custard. Essentially any dairy product.

C. Maltose – This disaccharide is formed from a combination of two glucose molecules. Maltose is popularly known as malt sugar.

Our bodies can utilize maltose as a source of energy, but we are not required to ingest large amounts of maltose in order to be recharged and energized.

Foods rich in natural maltose include sweet potatoes and kamut. Beverages such as ciders, beers, rice malt, and non-alcoholic malt-based beverages also contain this simple sugar. Syrups like brown rice syrup and barley malt syrup are also abundant sources of maltose.

3. Polysaccharides

Polysaccharides are sugar-based compounds composed of several simple sugars or monosaccharides connected together. These individual simple sugars are attached to each other via chains.

The most nutritionally important polysaccharides include cellulose, glycogen, and starch. Each of these compounds provides fiber and energy to the body.

Some of the polysaccharides, such as cellulose, cannot be digested by the body, however are important nonetheless in keeping the digestive system clean and healthy.

Glucose, galactose, and fructose are the three most common monosaccharides which can be found in polysaccharide compounds.

How Does the Body Process These Sugars?

The fast majority of the foods we consume contain sugars, although we may not be aware of it. Carbohydrate-rich foods are especially abundant sources of sugars, although these foods may not necessarily be sweet to the taste.

So what happens to these carbohydrates and sugars once they enter our body? Sugar digestion occurs in three main stages or places I.e. within the mouth, stomach, and intestines.

Mouth

Food gets mechanically separated into smaller pieces thanks to the chewing action of your teeth, tongue, and saliva. The salivary glands in the mouth release an enzyme called amylase to help break down your food into even smaller sugar particles. Since chewed-on food doesn't stick around for long in the mouth, amylase can separate only a small amount of sugar from the food being ingested.

This partially broken-down mass of food is technically called chyme. During swallowing, the tongue helps propel chyme down the esophagus and into the stomach.

Stomach

As chyme reaches the stomach, amylase becomes inactive due to the highly acidic environment here. The food gets further broken down by the gastric juices containing hydrochloric acid. Smaller molecules of sugar begin to break apart from the larger polysaccharides and disaccharides.

Food molecules remain here for around four to six hours. Even during this time frame, the stomach still cannot break down the food into the simplest monosaccharide sugars. The chyme eventually gets propelled into the small intestines for this to happen.

Small Intestines

The small intestine is the place where most of the sugar digestion and absorption takes place. This hollow muscular tube measures around 6 meters and is folded over with three distinguishable sections.

The small intestine contains the following structures and juices which help in breaking down the chyme and absorbing the sugar molecules into the body:

Digestive enzymes – these come from the neighboring organs, pancreas and liver. They break down food molecules into the simplest sugar forms (monosaccharides, especially glucose).

Glands - these secrete fluids which help neutralize the acidic nature of chyme from the stomach.

Villi – microscopic hair-like projections on the inner walls of the small intestine. They help in absorbing the sugars and other nutrients from digested food. They also propel undigested food down to the large intestine.

Now, as chyme enters the small intestine, it mixes with various digestive enzymes so that the monosaccharides can be isolated from the food molecules. Specific enzymes are used by certain sugars. The most common intestinal enzymes are the following:

- Maltase – breaks down maltose into two glucose molecules
- Sucrase – breaks down sucrose into fructose and glucose
- Lactase – breaks down lactose into galactose and glucose

Once these enzymes have successfully broken down the food molecules into fructose, galactose, and glucose, the villi alongside waves of muscular contractions, pushes them down to the mid section of the small intestine. This is where they are absorbed into the bloodstream and shuttled to the various cells of the body for absorption and energy consumption.

This is the fate of the digestible sugars we ingest each day. Simply put, they get mechanically and chemically separated into their simplest forms which the body can absorb and utilize.

Meanwhile, sugars which cannot be digested by the body such as pectin, fiber, and cellulose, continue their way through the small intestine and pass into the large intestine. Some fibers will be fermented by the resident friendly bacteria here, creating "good bacteria", the prebiotics which nourish the intestinal walls.

Glucose - The Daddy of All Sugars

Have you noticed that all the polysaccharides have glucose contained within them? Glucose is the most important energy-giving sugar available to us, which is why the fast majority of the foods and carbohydrates you will consume throughout the day provide ample amount of glucose within them.

Glucose gets absorbed into the bloodstream extremely easily after digestion. However it needs to be transported to the cells in order to be converted into energy or stored for future use. Glucose molecules float around in the blood, waiting for a carrier to pull them into the cells. And this carrier comes in the form as the hormone insulin.

All About Insulin

Insulin is an important hormone produced by the pancreas, a gland located behind the stomach. The pancreas has an abundance of beta cells, which are responsible for the production, release, and regulation of insulin into the bloodstream. These beta cells are highly sensitive and can readily detect the amount of glucose entering the blood.

Insulin secreted via the beta cells serves as a vehicle for sugar/glucose absorption from the blood into the various cells of the body. Without insulin, glucose would remain diluted in the bloodstream, where it could not be converted into energy nor stored for future use.

How Does Insulin Work?

Imagine the following: You've just woken one morning, and you suddenly eat a piece of fruit. Your digestive system breaks down the fruit into simple sugars and glucose. Then, these sugars will be absorbed into the bloodstream. The beta cells in your pancreas will suddenly sense this surge of glucose within the system, and immediately produce and release insulin to aid the glucose in getting up-taken into the bodily cells.

Insulin effects occur almost immediately. Glucose carrying insulin binds to insulin receptors at the walls of a cell. After which, the cell opens up and the glucose carrying insulin floods in. Glucose is now officially out of the bloodstream and inside of the cells, where it gets turned into energy. Any remaining unused glucose inside the cell will be stored for future energy production.

Insulin Sensitivity

This is where things get interesting (and potentially dangerous) with regards to sugar in excess amounts. Too much glucose in the bloodstream can lead to potentially fatal effects in the body overtime. This is why efficient insulin production and release is extremely important in regulating the levels of glucose in the blood, to keep them within a normal range.

Insulin generally lowers the amount of glucose in the bloodstream. How much insulin a person requires to keep his or her blood glucose levels in check, spells the difference in terms of insulin sensitivity.

Insulin sensitivity simply refers to an individual's level of responsiveness to insulin's effects. Some people may need to produce a small amount of insulin to regulate their blood sugar levels; these people have high insulin sensitivity. Others may require large amounts to see even a nominal lowering of blood sugar levels; these people have low insulin sensitivity. Something you want to avoid!

A Summary of Sugar

To cap it all off, sugar plays an essential role in keeping our bodies functioning and energized. There are many forms of sugar, but the main source the body requires is glucose. Our bodies have a simple but seemingly complex way of turning the food we eat into this glucose, which provides energy for everything from physical motor skills to mental arithmetic.

Therefore, there is indeed more to sugar than meets the eye. It's not just the food sweetener we're all so familiar with. Sugar is abundant in every carbohydrate-rich food, and it does so much more than simply make our meals taste pleasantly sweet.

However, consuming too much of the wrong type, and for extending periods of time, can be a BIG issue. Now that the dry scientific stuff is out of the way, the following chapter will outlines just how destructive this can be to overall health and well-being.

CHAPTER 3: HEALTH CONSEQUENCES OF CONSUMING TOO MUCH OF THE SWEET STUFF

"Pure white sugar, addictive and without nutrition"

(Marty Kaplan)

As we have seen in the previous chapter, sugar is an essential component when it comes to human nutrition. It's provides us with our main fuel and energy source to power our existence. But this certainly doesn't mean we have to consume super high amounts of the stuff in order to remain healthy. Quite the opposite. Too much sugar intake can harm your health in a myriad of ways.

Excessive sugar intake can make people sick. Like really sick. This is a widely-known fact, yet people continue to consume it in large quantities in their diets each day. However, it can be difficult to determine exactly how much you are consuming, as added sugar is in literally every prepacked and processed food on the market. Combine this with a small scoop in your coffee, a little syrup drizzled on your fruit, and you're starting to really exceed safe amounts.

In the second half of this book we will discuss the various means and ways of identifying these "bad" food groups and high sugar sources. We will also uncover the foods and recipes to stick by in order to eliminate unnatural and added sugar from your diet completely. But for now, we will simply take a look at the implications excessive sugar consumption can have on your overall health.

What Happens When the Body Takes in Too Much Sugar?

Here are some unpleasant changes which occur within the body when you consume large amounts of the sweet stuff for prolonged periods of time:

Metabolic dysfunction

Eating too much sugar-laden foods simply deposits excess glucose and fructose into the cells. The thing is, the body doesn't need all of this extra sugar for energy, it's overkill. Instead of being stored for future energy production, the metabolism functions in an abnormal way, leading to the production of stored fat from these additionally accumulated sugars.

Symptoms of metabolic dysfunction include weight gain, increase in abdominal girth, high blood pressure, high blood sugar levels, and an increase in bad cholesterol (LDL) levels.

Increased susceptibility to infection

Yeasts and bacteria commonly invade the human body, and these two organisms feed on sugar to grow and proliferate. Hence, an excessive sugar consumer stands a far higher chance of catching bacterial and fungal infections. The excess sugar circulating within the body encourages the growth of these disease-causing yeasts and bacteria.

Accelerates aging

Sugar can attach itself to proteins during a process known as glycation. When this occurs, the new substance formed from this synthesis can find its way into a person's tissues and speed up the loss of elasticity within them. Collagen and elastin fibers within the dermis layer breakdown and rupture, which can contribute to the appearance of sagging skin, a hallmark sign of physical aging.

Wreaks havoc on the liver

The liver is the only organ in the body where fructose, a type of monosaccharide, is metabolized. Excessive intake of fructose rich foods will certainly take a toll on the liver. Overloading the body with high sugar intake initiates this damage.

Tricks the brain into dependence and addiction

As we will see in the following chapter, sugar can be highly addictive. It stimulates the brain into producing our favorite feel good chemical, dopamine. Your brain becomes flooded with dopamine each time you eat sugar laden foods.

This eventually gives you that "craving" feeling until you get your hands on another sugary treat, to satisfy this sweet tooth and provide you with this pleasurable sensation once more. Being at the constant mercy of these sugar rush roller coaster mood swings is no way to live!

Causes tooth decay and cavities

Undigested sugar around your teeth and mouth are eaten up by bacteria which causes cavities, plain and simple. This paves the way for faster tooth decay and bad breath. Not good. It will also lead to more frequent, painful and expensive visits to the dentist…

Insulin resistance

Remember insulin, glucose's carriage from the blood into the cells? Well too much sugar in the blood for long periods of time can trigger your pancreas into continuously secreting large amounts of insulin, which in turn makes the body resistant to its effects.

The body is then required to produce insulin in greater amounts during a glucose surge, as the cells aren't responding to the existing and relatively large quantities of insulin already available. This will cause a build-up of stranded glucose molecules in the bloodstream, leading to chronic high blood sugar.

Insulin resistance is one of the precursors of diabetes mellitus and gestational diabetes. More on this now.

Illnesses & Disease From High Sugar Consumption

So we've now seen at a glance just how bad too much sugar intake can be on your body in the short term. But that's just the start. There are much more serious implications and debilitating conditions high sugar consumption eventually produces. Here is a rundown of the main illnesses you might develop if you don't cut down your excessive sugar intake pronto:

1. Diabetes Mellitus

This chronic and irreversible disease is probably the most well known illness resulting from excessive sugar consumption.

Diabetes Mellitus, or type 2 non-insulin dependent diabetes, may occur when:

- The pancreas produces insufficient amounts of insulin
- The body cannot use this insulin properly
- The bodily tissues have developed insulin resistance

All of these situations result in a glucose build-up in the blood. Elevated levels of sugar in the bloodstream can cause a variety of problems, including high blood pressure, nerve damage, kidney diseases, and eventually a stroke.

Symptoms of diabetes mellitus include the following:

- Sudden or unexplained weight loss
- Excessive thirst
- Frequent urination and urinary infections
- Uncontrollable and extreme hunger even after eating
- Weakness and fatigue
- Tingling sensation in the hands or feet
- Dry mouth
- Blurred vision

This illness has no cure, just management. Lifestyle changes, especially dietary modifications, are the key to living with diabetes in a comfortable way. Those with inadequate insulin production may benefit from insulin shots similar to those given with type 1 diabetes (wherein a person cannot produce insulin to begin with).

Medications to help the body react normally to insulin (such as Metformin) may also be prescribed to patients with diabetes mellitus. Of course you should always be under a doctors supervision when treating these conditions. However, my aim for this book is to hopefully prevent things from getting to this stage in the first place via dietary intervention.

2. Hypertension

High amounts of sugar in the bloodstream can make it highly viscous. This requires the heart to pump more forcefully into the blood vessels, so that the thicker, sugar-laden blood can pass through efficiently.

Diabetics often experience hypertension as a complication of their uncontrolled diabetes. Hypertension may lead to other fatal conditions such as heart attacks, coronary artery disease, and again, a stroke.

Hypertension can be a tricky one to spot too, as it may not present you with any signs and symptoms initially, other than higher systolic and diastolic readings on a blood pressure check. Medications to treat hypertension in people with high sugar intake or diabetes, include ACE inhibitors and diuretics.

3. Atherosclerosis

People who consume too much sugar are at risk for plaque build-up in their arteries, a condition known as atherosclerosis. Sugar, alongside cholesterol, calcium, and saturated fat, can accumulate in the walls of blood vessels to form plaque deposits. This plaque hardens overtime and causes a narrowing of the blood vessel's internal walls.

Atherosclerosis can be treated by lowering the consumption of sugar and cholesterol rich foods. Statin medications may also be prescribed to lower cholesterol levels in people with hypertension and diabetes, alongside atherosclerosis. But again, I always find that dietary modifications are your best bet for beating this stuff, certainly to begin with.

4. Alzheimer's Disease and Dementia

These two illnesses are characterized by progressive cognitive decline and brain shrinkage. They both lead to poor quality of life, especially in the latter years of ones life. Recent studies have shown links between excessive sugar intake and the development of these diseases.

It appears that high blood sugar associated with diabetes can weaken the small blood vessels in the brain. This leads to minor brain damage, which subsequently causes cognitive impairment. A similar build up of plague in these capillaries of the brain can restrict blood flow to certain areas, exacerbating this memory loss and cognitive decline.

Another possibility links the death of brain cells to insulin resistance. Remember that brain cells rely solely on glucose for nourishment? When a diabetic person develops insulin resistance, glucose will have no carriage to get through the blood brain barrier. Hence, brain cells diminish and they're not easily reproducible like the other cells in the body. If a brain cell dies, regeneration takes time and is by no means a certainty.

5. Polycystic Ovarian Syndrome (PCOS)

Women who consume too much sugar are at high risk for developing polycystic ovarian syndrome (PCOS). This endocrine condition occurs when the ovaries produce multiple matured eggs, but fail to release them. This leads to hard cysts appearing on the surface of the ovary. Ovulation is impaired as the eggs aren't released, altering the normal menstrual cycle. This causes irregular periods, and making conception hard to achieve.

Insulin resistance is once again PCOS's link to sugar. Blood sugar spikes due to insulin resistance. Hence, the pancreas is pressured into continually secreting more insulin, even if the body doesn't respond to it. The large quantities of insulin reaches the ovaries and triggers them to secrete more male hormones, which in turn overpower the female hormones. The end result is a disruption on the ovaries normal functions.

No cure has been developed for PCOS as yet; the infertility symptoms are the only ones being treated with hormonal therapy. But most women who are insulin resistant find that decreasing or even quitting sugar intake altogether, improved their symptoms and gradually resolved their PCOS, allowing them to become fertile again.

Preventing These Ailments

I have included this detailed overview of sugar and the adverse effects it can have on the human body, simply to make you aware of the damage you might be causing with a high sugar intake diet. To highlight the dangers that continuing down such a path can potentially bring. To scare you into some action here.

The key to preventing many, if not all of these illnesses is really simple. Cut down your sugar intake. Stop gorging on sweet snacks, chocolates, pastries, cookies, cakes, and fast food take-aways. In essence, go on a sugar detox!

CHAPTER 4: HUMANITIES DRUG OF CHOICE - ARE YOU ADDICTED?

"Sugar is eight times as addictive than cocaine"

(Mark Hyman MD)

I don't put sugar in my tea. I don't drink coke or eat doughnuts. But that is just the face value stuff. Sugar is laced within almost everything we eat these days. Usually hidden in salad dressings, condiments, nut butters, yogurts, white breads. Essentially anything processed. So you might not feel like you are addicted to this stuff, but dig a little deeper and you may be surprised at just how dependent you've become.

We have already discussed the major health implications here, but it is claimed that sugar (and its related side effects) has killed more people than alcohol and tobacco related deaths combined. There is still some debate as to what contributes to diabetes more I.e. high refined sugar or high saturated fat intake. However, they both certainly play their part and combining them is a disaster for your health.

Currently 40%-50% of Americans will develop metabolic syndrome, which usually leads to full blown diabetes. Whatever figure you deem to be acceptable, this is many magnitudes greater than it should be. Along with obesity, the annual cost of treating these diseases runs into the hundreds of billions ($182 billion - current estimate).

If you have either of these two conditions, you are also 4-5 times more likely to experience a stroke. Hopefully you are not at this point yet. The idea for this book is to halt this seemingly unstoppable march to ill health and an early grave, by preventing it from getting that far in the first place. So how do you know if you are indeed a sugar addict?

The Telltale Signs:

1. Do you instantly feel better when you eat sweet and sugary foods?

2. Do you instantly feel better when eating refined starchy carbs such as white breads & pasta?

3. Have you ever tried to cut back on these things and failed to do so?

4. When you attend dinner events and birthday parties are you unable to turn down the cakes & desserts?

5. Do you typically crash around mid-afternoon if you haven't had any sweet or sugary foods to "keep you going"?

If you answer "Yes" to most or all of these questions, than you are indeed addicted to this stuff. In reality, just about every person reading this will be. So don't be ashamed, I was also in this category for most of my life too. It's so prevalent and accepted in society today. It's not actually your fault for the most part. This stuff is pushed onto us so hard by big food producers it's almost impossible not to enter into this addictive cycle.

Current Guidelines

So how much sugar should we be consuming ideally? This is a difficult one to answer as we have already seen, sugar or glucose runs our entire biological machinery. A better question would be, how much refined or added sugar should we be consuming on a daily basis? What are the safe and recommended levels to stick by?

These figures are continually being revised downwards year after year which somewhat says a lot in its own right. The American Heart Association currently recommends around nine teaspoons a day (36 grams) for men. They suggest that six teaspoons (24 grams) is the upper recommended limit for women, with just three teaspoons (12 grams) for children.

However, the average American adult today takes in around 126 grams of sugar each and every day! This has been slowly climbing since the 70's. Nobody needs to point out that this is excessive. So how do we fix this endemic problem which plagues society in such a big way? We go on a sugar detox!

Preventing a high-sugar addiction takes a total lifestyle change. Make the necessary tweaks in your diet and incorporate healthy habits bit-by-bit into your daily grind. Discipline yourself to think in a healthier manner which will inevitably lead to a happier, healthier and ultimately more fulfilling life going forward.

The second part of this book will focus on just how to do this effectively. The chapters will outline the practical steps to beat this addiction once and for all…

PART 2: PRACTICAL WAYS TO ELIMINATE ADDED SUGAR FROM YOUR DIET (AND REPLACE WITH HEALTHIER ALTERNATIVES)

CHAPTER 5: GETTING OFF THE SUGAR RUSH ROLLER COASTER!

"Let food be thy medicine, and medicine be thy food"

(Hippocrates)

In a perfect scenario we want to keep our blood sugar as stable as possible, not too high and not too low. Maintaining a consistently high glucose level throughout the day puts unwanted pressure on the pancreas to produce ever increasing amounts of insulin, damaging the cells over time. If this continues, the body will become acclimatized to these high levels, making weight loss much harder to achieve and even leading to metabolic damage over time.

However, this is what many people are doing in order to stave off sugar crashes. They continually have to consume high sugar foods, to snack on biscuits and candies to fight the crash which inevitably comes in hours after eating such food sources in the first place. They have to prevent this lull in energy and motivation which comes from low blood sugar levels. Not a good situation in the slightest.

So how do we combat this? We stop our dependence on these food sources and we switch to added/refined sugar free, low Glycemic

Index (GI) whole foods. The GI scale simply reflects the effects at which carbohydrates contained within a certain food has on a persons blood glucose levels. Essentially the higher this number, the more quickly the sugars are broken down and enter into the blood stream, and vice versa.

So in order to get off this sugar rush roller coaster, it's essential to start consuming extremely low GI foods as your daily base nutrition. We will explore what the best sources of these foods are shortly. But first its important to identifying what we should be getting rid of. What you should be clearing out of the pantry and kitchen cupboards for good.

If you are confused about what these high GI, high added sugar foods are, then you simply have to look at the contents tab on the back of the packaging. As a rule of thumb, anything with ingredients including 'ose' or 'syrup' at the end, has to go! Dextrose, dextrin, maltodextrin, maltose, high-fructose corn syrup, brown rice syrup, refiner's syrup, carob syrup, cane sugar, caramel, agave, stevia are all big red flags.

Good Carbs vs Bad Carbs

What is a Zero Sugar, low GI Carb source?

Fructose containing fresh Fruit, vegetables, beans/legumes/lentils, unsweetened whole grains & cereals (brown rice, Quinoa, Oats). These foods take longer to break down, often requiring the decasing of seeds for instance, which ensures they are lower GI by very nature compared with regular flour.

Avoid sugary cereals in the morning due to high insulin sensitivity as this time (especially if your goal is weight loss). I talk at length about this within "Intermittent Fasting: A Nutritionists Guide". Eat plenty of oats, the simply ones which simply have one ingredient in them. Oats! Avoid the instant brands which come in the small flavored packages, as they are laden with sugar and sweeteners. Even granola or muesli with honey can put you over 26 grams in one sitting…!

What is a clean protein source?

Egg whites

Fresh wild caught fish, not farmed (Salmon, Cod, Sardines)

Lean poultry (chicken, Turkey breast)

Greek yogurt

What are healthy sources of fats?

Nuts (Almonds, Brazil & Walnuts)

Seeds (Flax, Chia, Hemp)

Avocado

Natural Oils (Olive, Canola, Grape-seed)

My number one rule is to essentially avoid anything which comes in a packaging of any kind to begin with. Go do your weekly grocery shopping and ONLY put these stated whole foods in your basket. Avoid sucrose packed fruit juices, milk, yogurt, honey & maple syrup. These types of food are way to nutrient dense with empty sugary calories.

I've heard people say things like "eating one medium sized apple is as bad as eating one packet (2 cups) of Reese's Peanut Butter Cups, as they both contain 21 grams of sugar". Whilst this is technically true, they are missing the entire point. The chocolate bars, biscuits and candy are empty calories. They are refined sugar and nothing else. They are designed to keep you on the sugar rush roller coaster...

Whole foods on the other hand, such as fresh fruits and vegetables, contain a whole host of health benefiting micro-nutrients such as vitamins, minerals and antioxidants. They also contain essential roughage and fibre to aid digestion. So now that you have a better idea of what exactly you should be throwing out, and what to replace this with at the supermarket. It's time to take a look at some specific meal plans and recipes to start your own sugar detox!

CHAPTER 6: ZERO SUGAR RECIPES AND ALTERNATIVE MEAL PLANS

"Your diet is a bank account. Good food choices are good investments"

(Bethenny Frankel)

The trick is to keep things simple, but substantial to begin with. You want to ensure you feel satisfied and that you are not missing out. This goes back to nutrient density and caloric composition of the foods you will be eating. Make these meal portion sizes around 30% larger compared with your regular, added sugar meals of the past. They will contain roughly the same amount of calories, so you will feel just as satiated after eating them.

Removing sugars from your diet is about minor adjustments, if you want the highest chance of success. It's about modifying your favourite foods with alternative ingredients and upping the plate size if you have to. Remember you are still able to eat unlimited vegetables, so pile your plate with the ones you love. This even includes sweet potatoes & beetroots. Just remember whole foods and back to the basics!

Also understand that it's OK to maintain or even increase your intake of proteins and healthy fats as you make this transition away from added sugar foods. The idea is to keep you as content as possible, to stave off any potential sugary carb cravings throughout the day. The following is a breakdown of my three go-to meals plans for each eating session of the day:

Breakfast

My favorite cooked option:

2 Eggs, whole-grain bread (toasted), spinach, cherry tomatoes and avocado.

- You can add smoked salmon and capers if you like.

My favorite smoothie option:

1 cup of oats, 1/2 cup of frozen blueberries, 1 frozen banana, handful of spinach, teaspoon of ground flax seeds, 1 scoop of vegan chocolate protein powder (from hemp, pea, rice protein).

- You can add 1 teaspoon of unsweetened peanut or almond butter if you like.

My favorite fruit option:

Broiled grapefruit or melon. Simply cut open the fruit and spray with some coconut oil, add a sprinkle of cinnamon powder and broil in an oven until charred. Then you are good to go!

Lunch

My favorite salad option:

Tuna salad with arugula, onion, green peppers, seeded crackers & cracked black pepper.

- You can add green or black olives if you like.

My favorite everyday option:

Steamed cauliflower rice with olive oil, garlic, lime juice, black beans, red peppers & seasoning.

- You can add lime zest/juice mixed with Greek yogurt if you like.

My favorite "junk" food option:

Chicken burger with avocado mayo, tomato, lettuce and sweet potato fries.

- You can add an additional side salad of your choice if you are feeling healthy!

Dinner

My favorite pasta option:

Seafood olio aglio with whole-wheat pasta, jumbo shrimps, muscles, mushrooms, chilli flakes, garlic and olive oil.

- You can add some homemade garlic whole-meal bread if you like.

My favorite rice option:

Chilli with ground minced beef, kidney beans, green peppers, chopped tomatoes, oregano, cumin and brown rice.

- You can add half a glass of your favorite red wine if you like.

My favorite substantial salad option:

Grilled chicken breast with a quinoa base topped with kale, broccoli, chickpeas & cherry tomatoes.

- You can add a s homemade soup of your choice if this is still not enough.

Dessert

My favorite choco option:

100% cocoa dark chocolate with a serving of fruit of your choice. I would recommend mandarins, mango, berry's or pineapple to sweeten the bitter dark chocolate.

My favorite fruit bowl option:

Sliced bananas with strawberries, raspberries, blueberries, kiwi fruit, oranges & grapes.

My favorite "versatile" option:

(I name this one the versatile option as I sometimes substitute it in for breakfast or for a pre-workout hit if I'm feeling tired).

Two pieces of whole-grain toast with banana slices, natural peanut butter and sprinkled cinnamon.

*Note: If you absolutely have to add a sweetener such as honey, maple syrup to begin with, then do so. But use it super sparingly and try to eradicate this after a few weeks (you will naturally find yourself doing this anyway as they will start to taste too sweet!).

Snacks

1. Handful of raw almonds or Brazil nuts

2. Cucumber and/or carrot slices with homemade hummus dip.

3. Any piece of large fruit - apple, pear, banana etc

(Avoid dried fruit though. They are essentially condensed calories in the form of exclusive sugar, just without much in the way of nutrients or roughage and fibre which whole fruits provide. It's a similar situation to refined oils in terms of saturated fat content. If you have to treat yourself, do it with some dried dates or figs once a week with coconut ice cream for dessert).

The idea for these meal plans is to let you know what I like and find most easy to prepare and consume each day. They are designed to give you an idea of what ingredients you can add to your dishes, although they are certainly not set in stone. Have a play with them yourself, experiment with your own favorite foods and combinations. Ultimately that is the way to keep things fresh and interesting. That will give you the highest chance of success in sticking with this.

I'm in the business of teaching folks how to fish, not giving them one to feed them for a day. I could give you a list of 10 different options for breakfast, lunch and dinner. But that would not only overwhelm most people, its overkill to begin with. Again, the key is to master 2-3 dishes you like for each meal time and stick with them to begin with. Then slowly expand on your culinary repertoire once you have beaten the sugary carb cravings once and for all!

Things to Keep in Mind

You will have to prepare these meals yourself to begin with. Don't be lazy, you have to learn the skill of preparing these foods, even if you are not already a somewhat competent cook. Don't worry, you don't have to be a master chef by any stretch of the imagination. You simply have to do it to ensure you know the ingredients which are going into your meals. To ensure nothing with added sugar creeps into the dishes.

You will then have to bring these meals to work or were ever you are during the day to begin with. Restaurant food is ridden with hidden sugar and it's extremely difficult to find yourself a 100% sugar free meal at these places. The same goes for family meet-ups and dinners. Make sure that you eat fully before heading out to these events so you can politely decline any food which is on offer there.

Remember that this sugar detox will be challenging at first. The withdrawals you will experience can lead to fatigue and headaches among other side effects in the initial couple of days. Just ensure you are eating considerable portions of the aforementioned meal plans and drinking plenty of water throughout this adjustment period.

CHAPTER 7: DRINKS & BEVERAGES - THE EASIEST WAY TO REDUCE YOUR SUGAR INTAKE

My original intention was to simply add this section on drinks & beverages within the previous chapter with the sugar free meal plans. However, over the years I have come to realize how important a persons beverage choice is with regards to reducing sugar & weight loss for that matter. It really is the low hanging fruit when its comes to cutting out the sweet stuff from your diet.

In truth, most folks simply do not realize just how much added sugar their favorite drinks contain. This is especially true when it comes to soda's. A regular coke (12 ounce can) contains 39 grams of sugar! The situation is similar for just about every soda brand on the market. I'm not simply trying to single out Coke here. Even iced lemon tea's contain a lot of added sugar unless you ask for none!

It's literally everywhere. Ever thought that buying that "healthy" sports or isotonic drink is the answer? Think again. I actually spent a few semesters studying the contents of these beverages during my undergraduate. They are all essentially made up from a mixture of the following three components, just in varying quantities. They do of course contain some artificial flavorings and other additives, but the big three are:

- Water - The base fluid for the drink.
- Sodium - To aid in retaining the water for hydration.
- Glucose - Yes sugar! For energy.

Now depending on the brand I.e. Gatorade, Lucozade etc and also the climate the specific drink was designed for (yes these are designed for athletes!). These factors will play a big role in the amounts of the above three components found in these bottles.

For example, drinks intended for those competing in hotter and more humid climates, will contain higher water and sodium levels as its more important to remain hydrated during these conditions above all else. The sodium actually tricks the kidneys into thinking that you are less hydrated than you actually are, so decides to retain more fluid in the body than it otherwise would. Clever right.

However, those drinks designed for cooler climates typically contain a higher percentage of glucose, as hydration is less of an issue. In this case the extra energy source is given precedence over hydration. So keep this in mind the next time you are feeling sporty and reach for one of the colorful "health" drinks in the supermarket fridge.

If you haven't just completed a 10k run or mammoth workout, or plan on doing so in the next 30 minutes... then put it back. In fact, sugar consumption around training times is one of the only times I believe it to be allowable. This is due to the body being about to burn these carbs off as energy substrates. Or replacing the liver and muscle glycogen you have just worked off post workout. Again, I talk in greater detail regarding general carbohydrate timing within "Intermittent Fasting: A Nutritionists Guide".

However in general, the regular person should simply cut out all of the above sugary beverage choices. Especially when initially attempting a sugar detox. Instead, replace these drinks with any combination of the following alternatives and you will notice a big difference in your weight and overall health as a result.

Healthier Sugar Free Alternatives

Water!

For most people, simply replacing every drink they consume with a glass of water, would literally halve their daily sugar intake. It would also provide them no end of additional health benefits such as clearer skin, better concentration and improved sleep etc. All this coming from elevated hydration levels. However, I realize this isn't always feasible as people do require some variance to stay the course.

Herbal, Green, Peppermint Tea (no sugar)

My most effective method of performing a sugar detox is with herbal teas. They are light on the stomach, taste great and give you a little caffeine boost to boot. Try not to overdo these. But if you feel yourself becoming tired or fatigued, especially during the afternoon, make yourself a cup of your favorite tea which should get you through until your next meal.

Black Coffee (no sugar)

If the herbal teas are not doing it for you, you have one more ace card up your sleeve. That is a strong coffee. Avoid sugar laden cappuccinos and the like. A strong black coffee should give you a large enough caffeine hit to squash any significant carb cravings. I know this is simply swapping one vice for another. But in the beginning stage of a sugar detox you have to do what you can to stay the course. Just fix one thing at a time!

Other Drinks to Avoid

Fruit Juices

You need to be cautious when it comes to juices. You have to be cognizant of your natural sugar intake for the day. I usually recommend no more than 2-3 servings of fruit per day during the first few weeks of detoxing. So one freshly pressed orange juice a day isn't an issue. But avoid cartoned fruit juices at all cost. They contain so much added sugar it almost puts them on par with full fat soda's!

On the days you are having fruit for breakfast or a smoothie, definitely refrain from any homemade juices and stick to water and tea that day.

Diet Drinks

Also avoid "diet" drinks and "zero sugar" beverages as they contain a lot of artificial sweeteners, such as aspartame & stevia, which are almost as bad as their full sugar counterparts. Studies have found that they may even promote weight gain to a similar degree compared with their sugar alternatives, not to mention a potential increased cancer risk too.

I used to drink Coke Zero as I thought I could use the caffeine hit without the calories. But I now simply opt for the herbal tea or black coffee options if I really need a pick me up. I would suggest you do the same. If you really are used to drinking these drinks and want to switch to "diet" version to begin with, then do so. But transitioning off of them as quickly as possible is the wise move to make.

If you really experience intense sugar cravings than make yourself one of the herbal tea's or black coffee first up. Then wait 30 minutes. If you are still experiencing the hunger pangs, then go brush your teeth! This may seem like a weird thing to do in the middle of the day, but it serves a clever little mind trick.

Nobody wants to eat or drink sugary things when they have the fresh taste of toothpaste in their mouth. You will find that your cravings will naturally subside when doing this, or will at least get you through until your next sugar free meal time!

CHAPTER 8: MINDSETS & HABITS - OVERCOMING ROADBLOCKS TO SUGAR FREE SUCCESS

"Success is not the absence of failure: It's the persistence through failure"

(Aisha Tyler)

The mind is undoubtedly a complex and powerful thing. But human cognition is a doubled edged sword. Having the ability to think things through in our minds is simultaneously a persons best friend and worst enemy. We can both contemplate past events whilst projecting future scenarios. This was essential for our development and survival throughout history. It was the mammals who could learn from their mistakes and plan ahead who would ultimately survive and thrive.

However, this advanced cognitive ability doesn't come without its downsides. Humans have a tendency to profess over many situations in life. Diet and lifestyle choices being no exception to this. It has been suggested that "over thinking" is actually the worst illness which plagues humanity today. If you are not careful you can get trapped in your own mind.

In general its best to quiet the mind for the majority of the day. However this is a far larger topic for another time. Lets just say that its beneficial to use your cognitive ability wisely, and simply to plan the necessary tasks you have to complete in the day. To organize your routines and eating habits before returning to relative calm and stillness in your thinking. This will help get you through some of worst roadblocks with regards to sugar detoxing.

There are many things which can get in the way of a healthy lifestyle, especially in the beginning when you are attempting to make the change. However, being forewarned is being forearmed in my opinion. The following are the three most important factors to prepare for when initially attempting to eradicate the sweet stuff from your day.

Mental Roadblocks to Watch Out For

1. Enlist a positive support group (or certainly one which won't derail you)

It's typically a good idea to recruit friends, family or colleagues when attempting to perform any major change in your life. You will be able to support each other and keep yourselves on track. At the very least, you want to be around those who understand what you are doing and support the efforts you are making.

Prepare for their responses when you tell them that you are going on a sugar detox. You will often get statements such as "Why are you doing that? Sugar isn't really a drug", or "the body cleanses and detoxifies itself naturally, you don't need to do that" and my favorite "You're already skinny, cutting out sugar will just be unhealthy for you".

2. You are worried that your actions might shame other people and hurt their feelings.

This is a genuine and common grievance people have. They believe that others will somehow be offended by what they are attempting. They don't want to put them through awkward moments at lunch or dinner times by being the fussy one in restaurants. Or they feel they are somehow being pretentious about their food choices and making others feel like they are making bad food choices.

This is something you simply must get over. It gets easier with age for sure, but you should never feel bad about improving you health. It will benefit you and everyone else around you immeasurably in the long run. Those who truly have your best interests at heart will support you and laugh off the nit-picking at social settings!

3. General fear of failure.

This is a big one. Most folks deem a sugar detox to be too daunting a task and shy away from it completely. As a result they never start down the path of cleaning up their diet, and suffer many of the health related consequences we've already covered earlier in this book.

Don't let this be you. Yes you might mess up on your first attempt at eliminating added sugar from your diet, but that's OK. You will learn vital information and gain experience on how to better implement it next time. Your chances of success will go up with every attempt. So don't let fear of failure prevent you from taking the first steps in the process.

New Habits to Cultivate

It is no secret that a person's daily habits and thinking routines will ultimately dictate how productive and successful they are. However habits are impartial, they will either help a person attain their desired results and remain persistent in pursuing them. Or they will ensure they continue getting the average/poor results they have always gotten.

So what are some of the most beneficial habits to cultivate whilst attempting a sugar detox diet? I touched upon a few of these in the previous chapter, however here is a full list of healthier sugar free habits which you should naturally find yourself cultivating, if you manage to perform a successful sugar detox.

Remember habits are actions we take each and every day, which add up into extremely positive and exponential results in the long run. This doesn't just apply to diet and lifestyle of course, but getting it right in this department is the greatest investment you can make in my opinion.

1. Having a much better grocery store experience

Spending the fast majority of your time in the fresh produce and organic aisles, is time well spent. It can seem overwhelming at first, but you will soon start noticing the difference between all of your favorite fruits and vegetables, as well as nuts and seeds. Upping your supermarket game is imperative to to succeeding at a sugar detox and is the first step on the road to success. It will also ensure that meal times are that much more flavorful and interesting. Which leads us onto habit number two.

2. Cooking with clean & fresh ingredients

One of the better habits I've picked up from cleaning up my diet, has been my overall cooking skills. Following on from selecting the right things at the supermarket, buying fresh also forces you to learn how best to cook them. Gone are the days when you will simply put a microwave meal in the oven for 5 minutes and be done with it!

You will have to learn to steam vegetables, broil fruit, stir-fry dishes. You will have to discover which herbs and spices compliment each other best, and the food combinations you like the most. This will become easier over time as your palate will become much more sensitive to the taste as your tongue is not constantly dulled down by overly sugary and sweet foods.

It will also help you better prepare food for the coming days, as nobody has time to cook every two hours. Simply cook enough food for another 2-3 portions which you can simply go back to the fridge for when its time for your next meal.

3. Eating whilst traveling

This is another big hurdle people find gets in the way of a sugar free and generally healthier diet. They can avoid those work lunches and social gatherings etc. However if you have to travel often, especially long distances, it can prove much more difficult. Airport food has improved a great deal in truth over the last decade or so. Before this it was almost impossible not to eat a Big Mac and fries whilst you waited for your flight, as McDonald's was the only restaurant in the departure lounge!

Nowadays it's much easier to pick up a healthy sandwich or smoothie juice for instance. Don't let yourself slip up on your diet when you travel. Long haul flights take their toll anyway, you might as well avoid the sugar rush roller coaster and get yourself some whole food, low GI substance before getting on the flight. You'll thank yourself in the end.

At the end of the day

Like anything else you want to change in life, its simply a matter of choosing to do this and committing in your mind. Honestly, this will be very personal to you, but if your "Why" is big enough, you'll find a way to see this through. If your intentions are weak however, you will inevitably fail.

So just go for it and see how it works out. In my opinion going cold turkey is the best way to go. It typically takes 3 days to get over the worst of the physiological discomfort which comes from removing sugar from your diet. It's no secret that you will likely feel like crap for a week or so, but its essential to break the habit.

It's also important to note that most people tend to store excess fat in this initial period as the body is adjusting and doesn't know what is happening. The lack of sugar makes the body panic and it starts to store even complex cards as adipose tissue, or certainly inhibits the release from existing stores.

So don't be disappointed if you don't lose belly fat straight away. The initial period is about adjustment, the weight loss and health benefits will quickly follow. They come in the weeks and months after this period. So stick with it as it will take more like 21 days to get over the psychological obstacles completely.

Studies show that it takes at least this amount of time for a new habit to become ingrained within our reticular activating system (RAS). The part of the brain which regulates our patterns of behavior.

SUMMARY

"Eating well is the most important act we can do to ensure health"

(Mark Hyman MD)

As I always ask myself when studying any exercise or nutrition concept, is there a body of evidence which supports this? Is there credible science behind why it should work? To make sense of it from a physiological standpoint. Then I see if this translates into practice in the real world. To see if I myself, and my clients are attaining the positive results the theory suggests we should be getting.

With regards to sugar detoxing, it's certainly no different. The health studies on consuming a low or no sugar diet couldn't be any more clear. Along with substantial anecdotal evidence which supports the positive benefits of this type of diet modification, from literally thousands of people across the globe. I certainly wasn't disappointed with the results when I went cold turkey on the sweet stuff nearly 3 years ago now.

In theory it should be an easy thing for people to take on board, a simply adjustment to make. Folks intuitively and logically know that added/refined sugar is bad for you, so usually don't need much persuading to take a stab at a sugar detox. However in practice, things can get much more tricky. Sugar has been ingrained so deeply into society over the centuries, eradicating it completely turns out to be a much bigger task when it comes to the crunch.

It begins with identifying and admitting your own addiction from the outset. Again, it's not about being ashamed here. 99% of the population will be in this camp to begin with. It's almost impossible not to be with regards to whats available to us at the supermarket and restaurants these days. It takes a massive conscious effort to undertake such a large scale dietary modification. Certainly to begin with.

But it will be so worth the effort in the long run. The list of human aliments suffered due to short term high sugar consumption such as inflammation, mood swings, fatigue and bad skin, is extensive. However, these pale in comparison to the more debilitative and dangerous longer term diseases and illnesses which come from prolonged high added sugar consumption.

Diabetes and obesity are such a bane on modern day civilization, its somewhat depressing to even glance at the mortality figures these conditions create. Insulin resistance and metabolic damage are no joke and we must do everything we can to avoid developing these conditions in the first place. Or at least lessen the impact on our lives if we do develop them.

This starts at the supermarket. It begins with a re-education on what you should be putting into your grocery basket each week. Essentially that should be anything your grandparents would recognize as "food". Whole foods and fresh produce. Nothing canned, processed or packaged to begin with. Yes, organically grown pesticide free products are a little more expensive (a lot more in some cases). But once again, you have to decide what is important in life.

It also includes what you should be throwing away, what you should be clearing out of your cupboards once and for all. This does take a lot of ingredient checking and label scrutiny at first. You want to avoid anything with more than 2-3 ingredients on the label. A can of tomatoes should include tomatoes, water and perhaps some sodium at most.

It should not contain countless chemicals and preservatives to ensure it has a long shelf life. With regards to added sugar contents, watch out for those "ose" additives or syrups of any kind. If you are buying fresh, this should not be an issue. Once you have got your supermarket game sorted, that's half of the battle won.

The next step is to begin practicing preparing your favorite sugar free meals. To experiment with what you like best and prepare enough to get you through each day. Remember things don't have to be dull and bland here. I have provided you with a base outline of ingredients and recipes I use on a day-to-day basis. Copy these if you like, or devise some of your own meals along similar guidelines.

Just remember that simple and substantial works best to begin with. You want to cut down your chances of re-lapsing with a sugary meal or snack as much as possible. So ensure you are eating big during this initial phase to avoid feeling light-headed and unsatisfied. Take your prepacked meals to work with you. In fact, take them every where you go for the first week or so. Restaurants will prove too tricky and tempting to negotiate during the initial 3 days of a sugar detox.

This is the most critical time, so do what you can to increase your chances of success. This will include enlisting the help and support of friends and family alike. Let them know what you are doing so they don't give you a hard time if you decline a social gathering or lunch with colleagues for instance. It will take at least 21 days to fully overcome the psychological bad eating habits, so stay as vigilant as you can during this time.

The true health and wellness benefits really take hold after this point. You will find yourself no longer craving the sugary foods, drinks and snacks you once did. Your palate will have completely adapted and it will be far easier to stay the healthy eating course. You will automatically pick up the fresh fruits and vegetables at the supermarket without the slightest feeling that you are missing out!

CONCLUSION

"Eat Less sugar. You're sweet enough already"

My aim for this book was to outline just how prevalent sugar has become in modern day society, along with the dangers that a high sugar consumption diet can have on overall health. However, I know this can be a difficult thing to achieve it practice. I certainly am not perfect in this sense, although I can now confidently claim that I have this sugar beast tamed once and for all.

In reality it's about what you eat for the majority of the time. For me that is now over 95% added sugar free, and I can't be more thankful that I have made the switch. There is a somewhat cliched phrase that "nothing tastes as good as health feels". But you really have to experience it to appreciate the validity of this statement.

Going sugar free has given me my life back in some sense. That may sound fairly dramatic to some, but it's the truth. I no longer have to eat that chocolate bar or biscuit during the day to keep me productive. I no longer have to consume the sugary drinks to keep me from crashing. Herbal teas and apples do the job so much more efficiently now.

If you haven't already tried to give this a go for yourself, I couldn't recommend it highly enough. You will likely fail the first time, but that's OK. Everyone does! It's about coming back the next time better prepared, which will give you a higher chance of success each time you get back on the horse. It's such a worthwhile goal to strive for.

I stand by the statement that good health is literally the best investment you can make in this world. Just think of how much more progress you can achieve with better concentration levels, improved sleep and the eradication of almost every human illness you can think of. Not to mention the hospital bills you will almost certainly be avoiding down the line.

So all I can do now is wish you the very best of luck on this health and lifestyle journey, especially if you are just starting out down this path. My suggestion would be to take the first step on a sugar detox diet, as that is the hardest one. Then everything else will begin to fall into place as you go!

All the best.

Simon

BONUS CHAPTERS

(From "Intermittent Fasting: A Nutritionists Guide")

CHAPTER 1: IT MAKES SENSE - THE SCIENCE BEHIND FASTING

"In a fast, the body tears down its defective parts and then builds anew when eating is resumed"

(Herbert M.Shelton)

The term intermittent fasting (IF) simply refers to the practice of not eating for extended periods of time throughout the day. As I mentioned within the introduction to this book, the concept is something that humans have been doing since our hunter gatherer ancestors inhabited the planet.

Today humans fast for a variety of reasons such as religious purposes, following certain rituals, food scarcity or simply sleeping. However regardless of culture and circumstance, the growing body of evidence and research is providing greater evidence to suggest that everybody should be partaking in some form of fasting throughout their day/week.

Hippocrates, the father of modern medicine, supported the practice of fasting and prescribed it to his patients. He suggested that, "To eat when you are sick, is to feed your illness." The same belief was held by other great thinkers throughout history, which include Plutarch, a Greek historian, Plato, and Aristotle. They all promoted fasting over the use of medicines.

"I fast for greater physical and mental efficiency"

(Plato)

It is part of human nature to stop eating when sick. This instinct is known as the physician within every human. If you have ever experienced over eating in the past, you will understand that it does more harm than good. A person tends to feel lethargic when full. Excess blood is directed to your digestive system and diverted away from vital organs including the brain. This is bad news if speed of body and mind is desirable.

So what are the reasons why so many people are reverting back to this type of lifestyle today? The two main considerations are body recomposition (I.e. fat loss/muscle gain) and the health benefits fasting can bring. I will get into these in greater depth within the following chapters, however here is an overview of both of these main benefits of IF:

#1 Weight Loss

IF helps you lose weight plain and simple. This process will naturally occur due to simply eating fewer meals. In addition to the reduction in overall daily calories, IF also boosts the hormones which aid in facilitating weight loss. As you go along with this style of eating, the levels of growth hormone production will also increase, as well as the concentration of norepinephrine in your system. You will also have lower insulin levels which will boost the breakdown of fats in your system. As your body gets used to the rhythms of IF, the body adapts and devises ways to use fats for energy more efficiently.

Even short-term fasting is effective in boosting a person's metabolic rate by up to 14 percent. This will allow you to burn more calories at a faster rate. A review of the scientific literature in 2014 found that IF is capable of helping a person lose up to 8 percent of his/her weight in just 3 to 24 weeks.

Another great benefit of IF is that the majority of the body fat a person will lose is around the belly area or the visceral fat. This fat is harmful as it builds up in and around the spaces of vital internal organs, such as the intestines and stomach. It produces toxins, including cytokines which reduces your sensitivity to insulin and increases your risk of heart disease. Cytokines can also worsen inflammation which increases your chances of certain cancers, especially those of the pancreas, colon, and esophagus.

Belly fat is a problem not only for overweight or obese people, but also for otherwise healthy individuals. This is due to the fat not only being stored as subcutaneous deposits I.e. beneath the skin, but also the internal organs as I mentioned above. However for most people aesthetics and physical appearance are the driving factor for wanting to lose weight (fat).

IF increases the propensity of your system to burn fat after it experiences a significant drop in the levels of insulin, and a boost in the levels of your growth hormone. The latter will also aid in building lean tissue which will further increase the fat burning potential of the person, as muscle is metabolizing energy substrates even whilst you sleep.

#2 Health Benefits

The first health component of IF is that it activates certain cellular repair processes, such as the removal of waste material. During the fasting period, your cells initiate autophagy or the "waste removal" process. As the cells break down, they metabolize the broken proteins in your body. When this process continues, your body will have more protection against various diseases, including most forms of cancer.

Cancer is a result of the uncontrolled growth of the cells. IF works by improving your metabolism, which results in a lower overall chance of developing such cancers in the first place. The studies done in this regard have largely been performed on animals, but the findings indicate promise for us too. Human cancer patients who follow the IF way of eating have shown a greater propensity to stave off cancer growth as well as reducing the effects of chemotherapy if they are undergoing treatment.

Another big consideration with regards to IF, is that it reduces oxidative stress, which is a major cause of chronic diseases. In fact oxidation is the only reason our bodies age in a physiological sense, and increased oxidative stress just speeds up this aging process. Although we can't escape this process, as oxygen is a critical component of the energy producing mechanisms within the cells, even when we are resting. However IF can reduce these levels as the person is consuming and metabolizing fewer energy substrates due to the overall reduction in caloric intake.

Essentially what is happening in the body during the oxidation process is the production of free radicals. These are atoms which are missing an electron is their out shell which can be highly destructive to the cells of the body. They will bump into healthy cells as they travel and steal these electrons to complete their structure, hence quickening the aging process and chronic disease formation.

You bodies natural defense system against this damage comes in the form of antioxidants such as vitamin C & E, which diffuse these destructive free radicals by donating an extra election in their out shell. This is especially important with regards to molecules in your system, such as DNA and brain tissue.

> "Intermittent fasting enhances the ability of nerve cells to repair DNA"
>
> (Mark Mattson - Neuroscientist)

IF is also highly effective in lowering insulin resistance and your blood sugar levels, which can greatly reduce your risk of Type 2 diabetes. There are studies which indicate that the fasting blood sugar of a person on this kind of diet, can be reduced by up to 6 percent, and fasting levels of insulin by 31 percent.

IF will also likely lower your risk of heart disease. It works by improving certain risk factors which include your blood sugar levels, total LDL cholesterol, blood pressure, inflammatory markers, and blood triglycerides.

As a result, it may also help prevent the occurrence of Alzheimer's disease. This neurodegenerative disease has no available cure, which makes prevention the key to delay its onset or reduce its severity. But it is likely a result of "atherosclerosis of the brain" meaning a clogging of blood vessels to the brain, very similar to that of the heart.

That being said, IF is also great for overall brain function. It boosts metabolic functions which affect the health of the brain in a positive manner. Animal studies have shown that it causes an increase in the growth of new nerve cells, attributing to greater overall brain capacity. These studies also found that this type of eating method protects the subject against brain damage after suffering from a stroke.

Fast Facts about Intermittent Fasting

To help you better understand some of the basic rudiments of the IF process, here are the most common frequently asked questions I get regarding this way of eating, and the answers I provide:

Is IF suitable for everyone?

The simple answer to this is, no. Whilst I believe (and the science shows) that intermittent fasting is perfectly safe and healthy for the vast majority of adults, there are some exceptions. You may want to avoid, or at least consult your doctor before starting an IF way of eating if you fall into one of the following groups:

- Pregnant or breastfeeding women
- You are under 18 years of age
- You have a history of serious mental health problems
- You are diabetic or taking medications for the disease
- You have recently undergone surgery
- You are suffering from a serious weight disorder
- You are underweight or malnourished

Should you exercise when you are fasting?

Yes, as we will see later on, it is actually important that you exercise during an IF program. Exercise compliments this style of eating very well, especially during the fasted state in the morning hours if weight loss in the goal.

Heavier resistance and weight training routines should ideally be performed later on in the day when adequate energy is available from the afternoon and evening meals. Again we will touch on the science and practical implications of this shortly.

Can you still undergo IF if you do not have an existing weight problem?

As stated above, IF offers many other benefits aside from just weight loss. This way of eating has a whole host of health/lifestyle benefits and is actually a very good way to develop self-control, helping a person maintain their current weight.

Does IF have any side effects?

The most obvious side effect of timing eating in this way is hunger, especially in the beginning when your body is still trying to adjust to the changes in your eating pattern. If you develop constant headaches and constipation, increase your water intake during the day. This should reduce your risk of experiencing any adverse side effects aside from hunger.

Does IF affect gout?

IF reduces inflammation, but again, make sure that you drink lots of fluid during the fasting hours. The condition can certainly worsen when a person becomes dehydrated. To reduce your risk of having gout or making it worse, avoid eating or consume a minimal amount of the following food items rich in purine: lentils, oatmeal, cauliflower, sardines, and liver.

How hungry can you get?

You will experience bouts of hunger to begin with, that's unavoidable. However you can counter this by walking, making yourself busy or drinking a calorie-free liquid. Coffee works best for me. When your body is receiving a reduced amount of calories compared to what its used to, it naturally boosts your metabolic rate. As time goes by, your body will get used to the hunger and you will know what to do to help yourself without breaking the fast. It does get easier I promise.

Why is it not advisable to those who have recently undergone an operation?

The important thing here it to give your body enough time and nutrition to heal. About 2 months for a major operation and a few weeks for a minor operation, before following any IF method. During the healing process, your body needs a constant supply of foods which are rich in micro nutrients and proteins to repair and rebuild. Whilst I have never seen adverse affects from anybody doing IF after such surgeries, it's always best to air on the side of caution until you are fully fit.

How do you maintain the weight you've lost through IF?

Once you have reached your target weight, it is recommended that you reduce the amount of days you fast per week. You can tweak the diet to suit your lifestyle. By the time you have gotten to this point, you will already be familiar with the right foods you should be eating and the proper techniques to control your cravings, to prevent yourself from overeating. Like everything else in life, discovering the best foods and times to eat them is a learning curve. Hopefully this book will give you a much better idea of how to get there.

How can you be certain that you are indeed losing weight?

It is your responsibility to monitor the changes in your weight. This is the only way you can be certain that your chosen IF method is working. However I would be careful of just monitoring the scales as the absolute measure of IF success. If you are exercising regularly you will more than likely be putting on lean muscle tissue in the process. This tissue weighs up to 3 times as much as fat, so you may not see the scales go down as fast or as much as you'd anticipated. But that's absolutely fine, as you are undergoing body recompositioning here, not just losing weight per se.

Measure your waistline as well as monitoring your weight on a weekly basis. You should find that the inches will start to fall off of the waist and hips most readily. However you may also want to measure your body fat percentage, because as I mentioned, metrics such as pure weight loss and BMI (body mass index) can be deceiving if you are gaining some lean muscle tissue in the process.

This can be measured at any doctors or health professionals office. Just about every main stream gym will now have a bioimpedance machine to calculate body fat percentage as well. Just ask one of the personal trainers if they have one to hand. I use them every week with my clients.

It is also a good idea to get them to check your resting pulse rate, blood pressure, levels of cholesterol, and fasting glucose if they can. There are devices which you can buy to perform these tests at home if required, or you can also have the tests done in a licensed clinic. This way you have a baseline reading for these metrics before you start an IF protocol. This will serve as a reference point in case you feel that something isn't going well when you do eventually start implementing a changed eating pattern.

CHAPTER 7: CARBOHYDRATE BACKLOADING

While the considerations of carbohydrate manipulation is a discussion in and of itself, in my opinion its one which ties in very closely with intermittent fasting. This is why I have included a chapter on carbohydrate backloading within this book.

Both strategies are essentially making best use of the bodies natural hormonal cycles and rhythms to aid a person in achieving their health and fitness goals, which is usually to get/stay lean whilst holding onto or building as much lean muscle tissue as possible.

I mentioned within the introduction that it was possible to have your cake and eat it with regards to weight loss, health and eating, if you know what you are doing. If you know how to time things correctly. I use a combination of IF and carbohydrate backloading to maintain an 8-10% body fat year round whilst almost eating what I want.

The key is carbohydrates and the timing of their consumption. Most people believe carbs to be the enemy, however nothing could be further from the truth. Carbohydrates are broken down into glucose and then glycogen, the number one substrate our bodies use to fuel everything, from movement to thinking.

The problem is when people consume too much, they begin to convert and store this excess glycogen as fat. However they need this carbohydrate energy source to get big and strong. On the flip side, a big reduction in carb intake will see the person lose weight, but find it very difficult to maintain and build muscle in the process (as well as always having a general lack of energy).

So how do you eat enough carbs for energy and muscle growth without putting on excess fat? Like IF, its about timing. More specifically its about insulin sensitivity timing. When you consume a carbohydrate heavy meal, the excess blood sugars trigger an insulin response and a signal for the body to uptake and store those carbs where it can. This will either be as liver/muscle glycogen or adipose tissue (fat stores) if the former are full.

So when is insulin sensitivity at its highest? There are two time periods predominantly. The first is in the morning when you first wake up. This is why I suggested that the inverted food portion pyramid works so well. Any food, and especially sugary or starchy carbs ingested at breakfast, will largely by absorbed and stored where ever the body can.

The second time when insulin sensitivity is high is immediately after heavy physical activity I.e. a resistance workout with weights for example. So taking this into consideration, how should you be timing your carbohydrate consumption?

As the name suggests, you need to be "backloading" these carbs in the latter part of the day. Avoid them in the morning when insulin sensitivity is high, if you are intermittent fasting this is not a problem as you are only drinking water or coffee. If you are carbohydrate backloading then you should only be consuming a high protein meal such as an egg omelette or protein shake etc.

The same should be followed at lunch time I.e. a high protein/ moderate fat meal consisting of foods already mentioned in the meal plans in an earlier chapter. This will again ensure no excess uptake of carbohydrates into the system.

Now here is the key. To make the best use of carbohydrate backloading, you need to make use of an afternoon workout. The most optimal time of day to do this is around 3-5pm when insulin sensitivity starts to wear off. However a heavy resistance type workout will actually kick it back into gear.

Now you have just had the benefit of working out fasted (which will burn excess fat) and it will also further deplete muscle glycogen stores which is the key to this working. After the workout you are free to eat anything you would like, including almost all of the sugary and starchy carbs you would like, up until bed time.

The reason you will not store any of these carbs as fat, even though you have just created a new insulin spike, is due to muscle glycogen stores being low or empty. So what the body does is shuttle these energy substrates straight back into the muscles to replenish the glycogen stores, ready for the next days workout. People will often find they can eat ice-cream, doughnuts, literally anything with this method and wake up the next morning even leaner than the night before! However I wouldn't advise this if you are sugar detoxing.

Now I know that it might not be feasible for everyone to workout in the afternoon, but it is possible to manipulate this a little by going to the gym in the early evening around 6-8pm. The concept still works.

The basic premise is to either consume no, or very few carbs in the morning/early afternoon before your workout, and load back up on them in the evening after your workout. Again much like IF, carbohydrate backloading works so well in that it not only runs alongside the bodies natural hormonal cycles, it also works with their lifestyle and social life patterns as well. It allows people to eat as much of and what ever they like whilst out for dinner with friends etc.

There is only one drawback to this way of scheduling carbs, which I have already touched upon within in earlier chapter, and that is having enough fuel in the system and energy to get a good resistance style workout in. I must admit, I sometimes struggle without any carbs before I train, so always add in around 30-50 grams for lunch on heavy training days.

However some people are OK to train just fine on zero carbs before working out. The carbs they eat the night before sufficiently loaded their muscle glycogen stores, which is the predominant fuel source you will be using during the workout anyway. On non training days, just follow a similar eating schedule I.e. little/no carbs until your evening meals.

They trick to all of this is to test these strategies out for yourself and see what your body responds to best. Then you can adapt things from there depending on how you feel and the results you are achieving. Whether that is utilizing a full IF program to eradicate all calories in the morning, or you are simply consuming proteins. The approaches are very similar in nature.

The premise is the same, stay away from sugary carbohydrates when either insulin sensitivity is high or muscle/liver glycogen stores are full. This will ensure that the body does not store these carbs as fat deposits on the body, but instead uses them to replenish energy stores in order to fuel your workouts.

Printed by Libri Plureos GmbH in Hamburg, Germany